Smoothies for Lowering Blood Pressure: Wholesome and Delicious Recipes

Healthy Eating

Table of Contents

Introduction

Welcome to a collection of wholesome and delicious smoothie recipes specially crafted to support individuals with hypertension in their journey towards better heart health. This book is a testament to the belief that taking care of our bodies can be a delightful and flavorful experience.

For those managing hypertension, making mindful dietary choices is crucial for maintaining balanced blood pressure levels. Smoothies, with their versatility and nutrient-rich ingredients, offer a fantastic way to incorporate heart-healthy foods into our daily routines. With the right combination of fruits, vegetables, nuts, and spices, these smoothie blends aim to nourish not only our bodies but also our taste buds.

In this book, you'll find a diverse array of smoothie recipes, each meticulously designed to pack a punch of essential nutrients, antioxidants, and natural goodness. From refreshing tropical escapes to cozy and comforting flavors, there's something to suit every palate and occasion.

Our mission is to empower you with knowledge and creative options, enabling you to take charge of your heart health without compromising on taste. By embracing these heart-smart smoothies, you can savor the joys of life while keeping your health a top priority.

Each recipe has been thoughtfully curated to incorporate ingredients known for their beneficial effects on blood pressure levels. We've carefully selected fruits, vegetables, nuts, and spices that offer heart-supporting properties, making these smoothies an excellent addition to your daily wellness regimen.

Whether you're already on a heart-healthy journey or just starting to explore ways to nourish your body, these smoothie recipes will serve as a delightful companion. Embrace the goodness of nature's bounty, and let these vibrant blends be a stepping stone towards a healthier and happier you.

Remember, every sip is an opportunity to nourish your heart, elevate your well-being, and revel in the journey of embracing a wholesome lifestyle. Cheers to your heart and vitality!

Recipe One: The Secret Garden Peachy Oat Smoothie

In the mystical realm of Mistwood, where ancient forests hide secrets of wonder and magic, a treasured collection of smoothie recipes has been guarded for generations. Each elixir holds the power to nourish not only the body but also the soul, enchanting those who Savor their flavorful mysteries.

One such concoction, known as "The Secret Garden Peachy Oat Smoothie," is a beloved favorite among the villagers of Mistwood. Its preparation is a dance of nature's finest offerings, blending the sweetness of peaches with the strength of oats and the creaminess of Greek yogurt. Let us venture into the enchanted recipe and awaken its magic:

Ingredients:

- ✓ 2 ripe peaches (fresh or frozen, peeled and pitted)
- ✓ 1/2 cup cooked and cooled oats
- ✓ 1 ripe banana
- ✓ 1/2 cup Greek yogurt (low-fat or non-fat)
- ✓ 1 tablespoon ground flaxseeds
- ✓ 1 cup water or unsweetened almond milk (adjust for desired consistency)
- ✓ Optional: Honey or a natural sweetener to taste (if needed)

Instructions:

1. Seek out the ripest and juiciest peaches, tenderly peel them, and remove the pits. These radiant gems carry the warmth of the sun within, adding a touch of magic to your smoothie.
2. In a pot, cook the oats until they reach a perfect texture. Let them cool, inviting the earth's nourishing embrace into your creation.
3. Combine the cooled oats with the ripe banana, Greek yogurt, and ground flaxseeds in a blender. These harmonious ingredients will work together to create a delightful symphony of flavors.
4. Pour in water or unsweetened almond milk to achieve your preferred consistency. Blend until all ingredients meld into a velvety elixir of refreshment.
5. Taste the smoothie and, if desired, add a drizzle of honey or a natural sweetener to enhance its sweetness, though the ripe fruits often provide all the sweetness needed.
6. Pour the Secret Garden Peachy Oat Smoothie into your favorite glass, and with every sip, let its magic nourish your body and soothe your soul.

In the realm of Mistwood, the Secret Garden Peachy Oat Smoothie is not just a recipe but a gift from the heart of nature. Each sip reminds us of the wondrous connection between the natural world and our own spirits. As you create and enjoy this enchanting elixir, may you feel the warmth of the sun, the wisdom of the earth, and the harmony of nature within every sip.

Recipe Two: Green Power Smoothie

Ingredients:

- ✓ 1 cup fresh spinach leaves
- ✓ 1/2 cup kale leaves (stems removed)
- ✓ 1/2 avocado (peeled and pitted)
- ✓ 1 ripe banana
- ✓ 1/2 cup Greek yogurt (low-fat or non-fat)
- ✓ 1 cup water or unsweetened almond milk (adjust for desired consistency)

Instructions:

1. *Prepare the Greens:* Thoroughly wash the fresh spinach and kale leaves under cool running water. Pat them dry with a clean kitchen towel or use a salad spinner to remove excess moisture. Remove any tough stems from the kale leaves.
2. *Blend the Powerhouse Greens:* In a high-speed blender, add the fresh spinach and kale leaves. These vibrant green powerhouses are rich in nutrients and will form the base of our energizing smoothie.
3. *Creamy Avocado Addition:* Add the half avocado to the blender. The creamy texture of avocado will not only enhance the smoothie's

consistency but also provide heart-healthy monounsaturated fats.

4. *Banana for Natural Sweetness:* Peel the ripe banana and add it to the blender. The natural sweetness of the banana will complement the greens and provide a delightful taste.

5. *Greek Yogurt for Creaminess:* Spoon in the Greek yogurt, which adds a luscious creaminess to the smoothie while also contributing protein and probiotics.

6. *Liquid Harmony:* Pour in the water or unsweetened almond milk to help the ingredients blend smoothly. Adjust the amount of liquid based on your desired thickness for the smoothie.

7. *Blend Until Smooth:* Secure the lid on the blender and blend all the ingredients until the mixture becomes silky and well combined. The vibrant green hue will indicate the richness of nutrients in the smoothie.

8. *Consistency Check:* After blending, check the consistency of the smoothie. If it's too thick for your liking, you can add a little more water or almond milk and blend again.

9. *Serve and Savor:* Pour the Green Power Smoothie into a glass and savor every sip of this nutrient-packed elixir. The combination of leafy greens, avocado, banana, and Greek

yogurt will leave you feeling energized and
ready to take on the day.

The Green Power Smoothie is not just a delicious
blend of flavors; it's a celebration of nature's bounty
and a true powerhouse of nutrients. As you enjoy
this invigorating beverage, remember that each sip is
a step towards nourishing your body with the vibrant
goodness of the earth's green treasures. Cheers to
your health and vitality!

Recipe Three: Berry Blast Smoothie

Ingredients:

- ✓ 1 cup mixed berries (blueberries, strawberries, or raspberries)
- ✓ 1 ripe banana
- ✓ 1/2 cup Greek yogurt (low-fat or non-fat)
- ✓ 1 tablespoon ground flaxseeds
- ✓ 1 tablespoon chia seeds
- ✓ 1 cup water or unsweetened almond milk (adjust for desired consistency)

Instructions:

1. Select Your Berries: Choose your favorite combination of fresh or frozen mixed berries. Blueberries, strawberries, and raspberries work wonderfully together, creating a symphony of flavors and colors.
2. Peel and Prepare the Banana: Peel the ripe banana and break it into chunks. The natural sweetness of the banana will complement the tartness of the berries.
3. Blend the Berry Medley: In a high-speed blender, add the mixed berries and the ripe banana. These vibrant fruits will be the star of the show, providing a burst of antioxidants and essential vitamins.

4. Creamy Greek Yogurt: Spoon in the Greek yogurt, adding a velvety creaminess to the smoothie while also boosting its protein content.
5. Nutty Goodness: Sprinkle the ground flaxseeds and chia seeds into the blender. These tiny seeds pack a punch of omega-3 fatty acids, fiber, and other beneficial nutrients.
6. Liquid Harmony: Pour in the water or unsweetened almond milk. The liquid will help create the desired consistency for your smoothie. If you prefer a thicker smoothie, use less liquid; for a thinner texture, add more.
7. Blend to Perfection: Secure the blender's lid and blend all the ingredients until the mixture becomes smooth and well combined. The vibrant hue of the berry blast will brighten your day.
8. Taste and Adjust: After blending, take a moment to taste the smoothie. If you desire a sweeter flavor, you can add a drizzle of honey or any natural sweetener of your choice. However, the natural sweetness from the ripe fruits might be sufficient.
9. Serve and Enjoy: Pour the luscious Berry Blast Smoothie into a glass, and savor the

explosion of fruity goodness with every delightful sip.

The Berry Blast Smoothie is more than just a burst of flavors; it's a celebration of nature's bounty and a delightful way to fuel your body with essential nutrients. As you relish the vibrant taste and color of this fruity concoction, remember that you are treating your body to a symphony of antioxidants and nourishment. Cheers to a berry-filled delight for your taste buds and your well-being!

Recipe Four: Beet and Berry Delight

Ingredients:

- ✓ 1 medium beet (cooked and peeled)
- ✓ 1 cup mixed berries (blueberries, strawberries, or raspberries)
- ✓ 1 ripe banana
- ✓ 1/2 cup Greek yogurt (low-fat or non-fat)
- ✓ 1 tablespoon ground flaxseeds
- ✓ 1 cup water or unsweetened almond milk (adjust for desired consistency)
- ✓ Optional: Honey or a natural sweetener to taste (if needed)

Instructions:

1. Prepare the Beet: Begin by cooking the medium-sized beet until it becomes tender. You can either boil it until easily pierced with a fork or roast it in the oven until soft. Once cooked, allow the beet to cool, and then peel off the skin. The vibrant color of the beet will lend a beautiful hue to the smoothie.
2. Select Your Berries: Choose your preferred combination of mixed berries – blueberries, strawberries, or raspberries. These

antioxidant-rich fruits will complement the earthy sweetness of the beet.

3. Peel and Prepare the Banana: Peel the ripe banana and break it into chunks. The banana will add natural sweetness to balance the flavors.

4. Blend the Beet and Berry Medley: In a high-speed blender, add the cooked and peeled beet, mixed berries, and the ripe banana. This medley of colorful ingredients will create a symphony of flavors and nutrients.

5. Creamy Greek Yogurt: Spoon in the Greek yogurt, adding a creamy and velvety texture to the smoothie while also providing an extra dose of protein.

6. Nutty Goodness: Sprinkle the ground flaxseeds into the blender. These tiny seeds offer a boost of omega-3 fatty acids and dietary fiber, contributing to the smoothie's overall nutritional value.

7. Liquid Harmony: Pour in the water or unsweetened almond milk to help blend the ingredients smoothly. Adjust the amount of liquid based on your desired thickness for the smoothie.

8. Blend to a Vibrant Fusion: Secure the blender's lid and blend all the ingredients until they fuse into a silky and visually

enticing delight. The harmonious blend of colors will be a feast for the eyes.

9. Taste and Adjust: After blending, take a moment to taste the Beet and Berry Delight. If you prefer it sweeter, you can add a drizzle of honey or your favorite natural sweetener. However, the sweetness from the ripe fruits may be sufficient.

10. Serve and Relish: Pour the captivating Beet and Berry Delight into a glass and relish each sip of this nutritious concoction. Embrace the nutritional power of beets and berries in a single, delightful package.

The Beet and Berry Delight is not just a delicious blend of flavors; it's a wholesome treat for your body and a celebration of the rich colors and flavors of nature. As you enjoy this vibrant and nutrient-packed elixir, savor the unique combination of earthy sweetness and fruity tang that will awaken your senses and nourish your well-being. Cheers to the delightful harmony of beets and berries!

Recipe Five: Tropical Paradise Smoothie

Ingredients:

- ✓ 1 cup fresh pineapple chunks
- ✓ 1/2 cup fresh mango chunks
- ✓ 1 ripe banana
- ✓ 1/2 cup unsweetened shredded coconut
- ✓ 1 tablespoon chia seeds
- ✓ 1 cup coconut water or unsweetened coconut milk (adjust for desired consistency)
- ✓ Optional: Honey or a natural sweetener to taste (if needed)
- ✓ Ice cubes (optional, for a chilled smoothie)

Instructions:

1. Prepare the Tropical Fruits: Start by cutting the fresh pineapple and mango into bite-sized chunks. The vibrant colors and tropical sweetness of these fruits will transport you to an island paradise.
2. Peel and Prepare the Banana: Peel the ripe banana and break it into chunks. The banana will add a creamy texture and natural sweetness to the smoothie.
3. Add a Tropical Twist: Sprinkle the unsweetened shredded coconut into the blender. The coconut's tropical aroma and

nutty flavor will infuse the smoothie with a touch of exotic paradise.

4. Seeds of Goodness: Add the chia seeds to the mix. These tiny seeds are rich in omega-3 fatty acids and dietary fiber, providing a nutritious boost to the smoothie.

5. Liquid Bliss: Pour in the coconut water or unsweetened coconut milk. This luscious liquid will bind all the tropical ingredients together and enhance the smoothie's tropical flavor.

6. Blend to Tropical Bliss: Secure the blender's lid and blend all the ingredients until they transform into a velvety tropical delight. If you prefer a chilled smoothie, you can add a few ice cubes before blending.

7. Taste and Enhance: After blending, taste the Tropical Paradise Smoothie. If you desire a sweeter flavor, you can add a drizzle of honey or your favorite natural sweetener. However, the sweetness from the ripe fruits is often sufficient to tantalize your taste buds.

8. Serve and Escape: Pour the tropical elixir into a glass and allow yourself to be transported to a paradise of flavors with every sip.

The Tropical Paradise Smoothie is more than just a blend of fruits; it's a delightful escape to a sunny oasis. As you enjoy the enchanting flavors and aromas of this tropical concoction, savor the essence of pineapple, mango, and coconut dancing in harmony. Let this smoothie become your ticket to a refreshing moment of pure bliss amidst the hustle of everyday life. Cheers to the tropical paradise in your glass!

Recipe Six: Watermelon Wonder Smoothie

Ingredients:

- ✓ 2 cups fresh watermelon chunks (seedless)
- ✓ 1 cup cucumber chunks (peeled and seeds removed)
- ✓ 6-8 fresh mint leaves
- ✓ 1 tablespoon fresh lime juice
- ✓ 1 cup coconut water or water
- ✓ Ice cubes (optional, for a chilled smoothie)

Instructions:

1. Prepare the Refreshing Watermelon: Begin by cutting the fresh watermelon into juicy chunks, ensuring that it is seedless. The watermelon's natural sweetness and hydration will be the star of this delightful smoothie.
2. Cooling Cucumber Addition: Peel the cucumber and remove the seeds before cutting it into chunks. The cucumber's crisp and refreshing flavor will complement the watermelon, making this smoothie a hydrating treat.
3. A Touch of Minty Freshness: Tear the fresh mint leaves and add them to the blender. The

mint will infuse the smoothie with a burst of invigorating and cooling freshness.

4. A Zest of Lime: Squeeze the fresh lime juice into the blender. The lime's zesty tang will elevate the flavors and add a hint of citrusy brightness to the smoothie.

5. Liquid Bliss: Pour in the coconut water or water to help the ingredients blend smoothly. Coconut water will enhance the tropical feel, while regular water will keep it light and simple.

6. Chill It Down: For a refreshingly chilled smoothie, you can add a few ice cubes to the blender before blending. This will make the Watermelon Wonder Smoothie even more enticing on a hot day.

7. Blend to a Luscious Blend: Secure the blender's lid and blend all the ingredients until they fuse into a luscious, pink-hued wonder. The aroma of watermelon, cucumber, mint, and lime will tantalize your senses.

8. Taste and Adjust: After blending, take a moment to taste the Watermelon Wonder Smoothie. If you desire a sweeter flavor, you can add a drizzle of honey or your favorite natural sweetener. However, the natural

sweetness of the watermelon is often enough to satisfy your taste buds.

9. Serve and Savor: Pour the refreshing elixir into a glass and savor every sip of this hydrating and invigorating concoction.

The Watermelon Wonder Smoothie is more than just a blend of fruits and herbs; it's a cool oasis on a scorching day. As you enjoy the blissful flavors and soothing aromas of this refreshing creation, let the hydrating power of watermelon and cucumber rejuvenate your body and mind. Whether you're seeking a moment of relaxation or a burst of energy, this smoothie is the perfect companion. Cheers to the wonder of watermelon!

Recipe Seven: Carrot and Orange Zest Smoothie

Ingredients:

- ✓ 2 large carrots (peeled and chopped)
- ✓ 2 oranges (peeled and segmented)
- ✓ 1 ripe banana
- ✓ 1/2 cup Greek yogurt (low-fat or non-fat)
- ✓ 1 tablespoon honey or maple syrup (adjust for desired sweetness)
- ✓ 1/2 teaspoon grated orange zest
- ✓ 1 cup water or orange juice (adjust for desired consistency)
- ✓ Ice cubes (optional, for a chilled smoothie)

Instructions:

1. Prepare the Vibrant Carrots: Start by peeling the large carrots and chopping them into smaller chunks. The vibrant orange hue of the carrots will brighten up your smoothie and add a dose of beta-carotene goodness.
2. Zest Up the Oranges: Grate the zest from one of the oranges using a fine grater or zester. The orange zest will infuse the smoothie with a burst of citrusy aroma and flavor.

3. Citrusy Segments: Peel the two oranges, removing all the white pith, and separate the segments. The juicy and tangy orange segments will be the highlight of this zesty concoction.

4. Creamy Banana Addition: Peel the ripe banana and break it into chunks. The banana will provide a creamy texture and natural sweetness to balance the flavors.

5. Velvety Greek Yogurt: Spoon in the Greek yogurt, adding a velvety creaminess to the smoothie while also boosting its protein content.

6. A Touch of Sweetness: Drizzle honey or maple syrup into the blender. Adjust the amount based on your desired level of sweetness. The natural sweetness from the fruits might be enough, but the honey or maple syrup can enhance the overall flavor.

7. Citrusy Zest: Add the grated orange zest into the mix. This addition will elevate the citrusy profile of the smoothie, making each sip vibrant and refreshing.

8. Liquid Harmony: Pour in the water or orange juice. The liquid will help blend the ingredients smoothly. Adjust the amount of liquid based on your preferred consistency.

9. Chill It Down: For a cool and refreshing smoothie, you can add a few ice cubes to the blender before blending. This is perfect for a revitalizing treat on a warm day.

10. Blend to a Zesty Fusion: Secure the blender's lid and blend all the ingredients until they combine into a smooth and citrusy delight.

11. Taste and Enhance: After blending, taste the Carrot and Orange Zest Smoothie. Adjust sweetness or citrusy flavor as needed to suit your taste preferences.

12. Serve and Delight: Pour the zesty elixir into a glass and enjoy the harmonious blend of carrots and oranges in every invigorating sip.

The Carrot and Orange Zest Smoothie is more than just a blend of fruits and vegetables; it's a zesty and revitalizing experience. As you relish the refreshing flavors and aromatic zest of this vibrant creation, embrace the healthful benefits of carrots and the zing of oranges. Let this smoothie be your delightful and nutritious escape into a world of citrusy bliss. Cheers to the zestful combination of carrots and oranges!

Recipe Eight: Creamy Avocado Delight

Ingredients:

- ✓ 1 ripe avocado
- ✓ 1 ripe banana
- ✓ 1 cup spinach leaves (fresh or frozen)
- ✓ 1 tablespoon almond butter (or any nut butter of your choice)
- ✓ 1 cup unsweetened almond milk (or any milk of your choice)
- ✓ 1 tablespoon honey or maple syrup (adjust for desired sweetness)
- ✓ 1/2 teaspoon vanilla extract
- ✓ Ice cubes (optional, for a chilled smoothie)

Instructions:

1. Scoop Out the Avocado: Begin by cutting the ripe avocado in half. Remove the pit and scoop out the creamy flesh into the blender. Avocado will provide a luxurious and silky texture to the smoothie.
2. Peel and Prepare the Banana: Peel the ripe banana and add it to the blender. The banana will contribute natural sweetness and a delightful flavor to the creamy concoction.

3. Nutrient-Rich Spinach: Add the fresh or frozen spinach leaves to the mix. Spinach is a nutritional powerhouse, adding vitamins and minerals to the smoothie while keeping it gorgeously green.

4. A Dollop of Nut Butter: Spoon in the almond butter (or any nut butter of your choice). The nut butter will enrich the smoothie with healthy fats and a delightful nutty taste.

5. Creamy Liquid: Pour in the unsweetened almond milk (or any milk of your choice). The milk will provide the creamy base for the smoothie, balancing out the richness of the avocado.

6. A Touch of Sweetness: Drizzle honey or maple syrup into the blender to enhance the sweetness. Adjust the amount based on your desired level of sweetness.

7. A Hint of Vanilla: Add the vanilla extract to the mix. The vanilla will add a lovely aroma and depth of flavor to the creamy blend.

8. Chill It Down: For a refreshing and cool smoothie, you can add a few ice cubes to the blender before blending.

9. Blend to Creamy Perfection: Secure the blender's lid and blend all the ingredients until they merge into a velvety and creamy delight.

10. Taste and Enhance: After blending, taste the Creamy Avocado Delight. Adjust sweetness or flavors as needed to suit your taste preferences.
11. Serve and Savor: Pour the luscious elixir into a glass and indulge in the creamy avocado goodness with every delightful sip.

The Creamy Avocado Delight is more than just a blend of fruits and greens; it's a luxurious and wholesome treat. As you savor the rich and velvety flavors of this creamy creation, appreciate the nourishing benefits of avocado and spinach. Let this smoothie be your delightful escape into a world of creamy indulgence. Cheers to the creamy goodness of avocado!

Recipe Nine: Cinnamon Apple Crunch Smoothie

Ingredients:

- ✓ 2 medium-sized apples (cored and chopped)
- ✓ 1 ripe banana
- ✓ 1/2 cup rolled oats
- ✓ 1 cup unsweetened almond milk (or any milk of your choice)
- ✓ 1 tablespoon almond butter (or any nut butter of your choice)
- ✓ 1 teaspoon ground cinnamon
- ✓ 1 tablespoon honey or maple syrup (adjust for desired sweetness)
- ✓ 1/4 cup granola (for topping)

Instructions:

1. Prepare the Apples: Begin by coring and chopping the medium-sized apples. You can leave the skin on for added nutrition and texture. The sweet and crisp apples will lend a delightful flavor to the smoothie.
2. Peel and Prepare the Banana: Peel the ripe banana and add it to the blender. The banana will provide natural sweetness and creaminess to the smoothie.

3. Hearty Rolled Oats: Add the rolled oats to the blender. The oats will add a delightful nutty taste and make the smoothie more filling and satisfying.
4. Creamy Nut Butter: Spoon in the almond butter (or any nut butter of your choice). The nut butter will add a creamy texture and enhance the nutty flavor of the smoothie.
5. Spice It Up: Sprinkle the ground cinnamon into the blender. The warm and comforting spice will give the smoothie a cozy and aromatic touch.
6. Sweetness of Your Choice: Drizzle honey or maple syrup into the blender to enhance the sweetness. Adjust the amount based on your desired level of sweetness.
7. Creamy Liquid: Pour in the unsweetened almond milk (or any milk of your choice). The milk will create a creamy and smooth consistency for the smoothie.
8. Blend to a Crunchy Fusion: Secure the blender's lid and blend all the ingredients until they combine into a smooth and satisfying blend with a touch of crunch from the oats.
9. Taste and Enhance: After blending, taste the Cinnamon Apple Crunch Smoothie. Adjust

sweetness or flavors as needed to suit your taste preferences.

10. Serve and Add Crunch: Pour the delectable blend into a glass and top it with a generous sprinkle of granola. The granola will add a delightful crunch and a wholesome touch to the smoothie.

11. Savor the Cinnamon Apple Crunch: Grab a straw and savor every sip of this comforting and crunchy creation.

The Cinnamon Apple Crunch Smoothie is more than just a blend of fruits and oats; it's a wholesome and satisfying treat. As you relish the cozy flavors and delightful crunch of this delightful creation, embrace the goodness of apples, oats, and cinnamon coming together in harmony. Let this smoothie be your comforting escape into a world of warmth and nourishment. Cheers to the delightful crunch of Cinnamon Apple Crunch!

Recipe Ten: Pomegranate Berry Blend Smoothie

Ingredients:

- ✓ 1 cup fresh or frozen mixed berries (blueberries, strawberries, or raspberries)
- ✓ 1/2 cup pomegranate seeds
- ✓ 1 ripe banana
- ✓ 1 cup unsweetened pomegranate juice
- ✓ 1/2 cup Greek yogurt (low-fat or non-fat)
- ✓ 1 tablespoon honey or maple syrup (adjust for desired sweetness)
- ✓ 1 tablespoon chia seeds
- ✓ Ice cubes (optional, for a chilled smoothie)

Instructions:

1. Select Your Berries: Choose your favorite combination of fresh or frozen mixed berries. Blueberries, strawberries, and raspberries work wonderfully together, providing a burst of color and antioxidants.
2. Prep the Pomegranate: Extract the pomegranate seeds from a fresh pomegranate or use pre-packaged seeds. The ruby-like pomegranate seeds will add a tangy and juicy pop to the smoothie.

3. Peel and Prepare the Banana: Peel the ripe banana and add it to the blender. The banana will add natural sweetness and a creamy texture to the smoothie.
4. Juicy Pomegranate Juice: Pour in the unsweetened pomegranate juice. The juice will amplify the pomegranate flavor and enhance the smoothie's vibrant color.
5. Creamy Greek Yogurt: Spoon in the Greek yogurt, adding a luscious creaminess to the smoothie while also providing protein and probiotics.
6. A Touch of Sweetness: Drizzle honey or maple syrup into the blender to enhance the sweetness. Adjust the amount based on your desired level of sweetness.
7. Nutty Goodness: Add the chia seeds to the mix. These tiny seeds are rich in omega-3 fatty acids and dietary fiber, offering a nutritional boost to the smoothie.
8. Chill It Down: For a refreshing and cool smoothie, you can add a few ice cubes to the blender before blending.
9. Blend to a Luscious Fusion: Secure the blender's lid and blend all the ingredients until they merge into a luscious and visually enticing blend.

10. Taste and Adjust: After blending, take a moment to taste the Pomegranate Berry Blend Smoothie. Adjust sweetness or flavors as needed to suit your taste preferences.
11. Serve and Savor: Pour the delightful elixir into a glass and savor the refreshing and tangy sweetness in every invigorating sip.

The Pomegranate Berry Blend Smoothie is more than just a blend of fruits and seeds; it's a burst of tangy and nutritious goodness. As you enjoy the delightful combination of berries and pomegranate, relish the vibrant colors and flavors coming together in this antioxidant-rich smoothie. Let this smoothie be your delicious and refreshing escape into a world of juicy delights. Cheers to the joyous blend of Pomegranate Berry Blend!

Recipe Eleven: Melon Mint Medley Smoothie

Ingredients:

- ✓ 2 cups cubed fresh melon (cantaloupe, honeydew, or a mix of both)
- ✓ 1 cup cubed cucumber (peeled and seeds removed)
- ✓ 6-8 fresh mint leaves
- ✓ 1 tablespoon fresh lime juice
- ✓ 1 tablespoon honey or maple syrup (adjust for desired sweetness)
- ✓ 1 cup coconut water or water (adjust for desired consistency)
- ✓ Ice cubes (optional, for a chilled smoothie)

Instructions:

1. Cube the Melon and Cucumber: Start by cutting the fresh melon into bite-sized cubes. You can use cantaloupe, honeydew, or a combination of both for a delightful melon medley. Next, peel the cucumber and remove the seeds before cutting it into cubes.
2. Minty Freshness: Tear the fresh mint leaves and add them to the blender. The mint will

impart a refreshing and invigorating flavor to the smoothie.

3. Zesty Lime: Squeeze the fresh lime juice into the blender. The lime's zesty tang will brighten up the flavors and add a hint of citrusy freshness.
4. Natural Sweetness: Drizzle honey or maple syrup into the blender to enhance the sweetness. Adjust the amount based on your desired level of sweetness. The natural sweetness of the melon and cucumber might be sufficient.
5. Cooling Liquid: Pour in the coconut water or water to help the ingredients blend smoothly. Coconut water will add a tropical touch, while regular water will keep it light and simple.
6. Chill It Down: For a refreshing and cool smoothie, you can add a few ice cubes to the blender before blending. This is perfect for a revitalizing treat on a warm day.
7. Blend to a Melon Mint Fusion: Secure the blender's lid and blend all the ingredients until they combine into a smooth and vibrant medley.
8. Taste and Enhance: After blending, take a moment to taste the Melon Mint Medley

Smoothie. Adjust sweetness or flavors as needed to suit your taste preferences.

9. Serve and Savor: Pour the refreshing elixir into a glass and savor the delightful combination of melon, cucumber, and mint in every invigorating sip.

The Melon Mint Medley Smoothie is more than just a blend of fruits and herbs; it's a refreshing and hydrating treat. As you relish the juicy sweetness and minty freshness of this delightful creation, embrace the hydrating power of melon and cucumber. Let this smoothie be your revitalizing and flavorful escape into a world of refreshing delights. Cheers to the refreshing fusion of Melon Mint Medley!

Recipe Twelve: Kiwi Lime Refresher

Ingredients:

- ✓ 3 ripe kiwis (peeled and chopped)
- ✓ 1 lime (juiced)
- ✓ 1 tablespoon honey or maple syrup (adjust for desired sweetness)
- ✓ 1 cup coconut water or water
- ✓ 1 cup ice cubes
- ✓ Fresh mint leaves for garnish (optional)

Instructions:

1. Prep the Kiwis: Start by peeling the ripe kiwis and chopping them into small pieces. The sweet and tangy kiwi will be the star of this refreshing smoothie.
2. Zesty Lime Juice: Squeeze the juice from the lime into the blender. The lime's zesty tang will enhance the flavor and provide a burst of citrusy freshness.
3. A Touch of Sweetness: Drizzle honey or maple syrup into the blender to enhance the sweetness. Adjust the amount based on your desired level of sweetness. The natural sweetness of the kiwi might be sufficient.

4. Hydrating Liquid: Pour in the coconut water or water to help the ingredients blend smoothly. Coconut water will add a tropical twist, while regular water will keep it light and simple.
5. Chill It Down: Add the ice cubes to the blender. The ice will cool down the smoothie and make it wonderfully refreshing.
6. Blend to a Luscious Refresher: Secure the blender's lid and blend all the ingredients until they combine into a smooth and revitalizing refresher.
7. Taste and Adjust: After blending, take a moment to taste the Kiwi Lime Refresher. Adjust sweetness or flavors as needed to suit your taste preferences.
8. Serve and Garnish: Pour the refreshing elixir into a glass and garnish with fresh mint leaves, if desired. The mint leaves will add an extra touch of coolness and aromatic delight.
9. Sip and Refresh: Grab a straw and savor every sip of this invigorating and revitalizing creation.

The Kiwi Lime Refresher is more than just a blend of fruits and lime; it's a zesty and hydrating delight. As you enjoy the tangy sweetness and citrusy freshness of this refreshing creation, embrace the goodness of kiwi and lime. Let this smoothie be your energizing and revitalizing escape into a world of delightful flavors. Cheers to the rejuvenating fusion of Kiwi Lime Refresher!

Recipe Thirteen: Papaya Passion Smoothie

Ingredients:

- ✓ 1 ripe papaya (peeled, seeds removed, and chopped)
- ✓ 1 cup fresh pineapple chunks
- ✓ 1 ripe banana
- ✓ 1/2 cup Greek yogurt (low-fat or non-fat)
- ✓ 1 tablespoon honey or maple syrup (adjust for desired sweetness)
- ✓ 1 cup coconut water or orange juice (adjust for desired consistency)
- ✓ 1/2 teaspoon grated fresh ginger (optional, for a zesty kick)
- ✓ Ice cubes (optional, for a chilled smoothie)
- ✓ Fresh mint leaves for garnish (optional)

Instructions:

1. Prep the Papaya: Start by peeling the ripe papaya and removing the seeds. Chop the papaya flesh into small pieces. The sweet and tropical papaya will be the star of this exotic smoothie.
2. Pineapple Punch: Add the fresh pineapple chunks to the blender. Pineapple's tangy

sweetness will complement the papaya, creating a delightful tropical blend.

3. Peel and Prepare the Banana: Peel the ripe banana and break it into chunks. The banana will provide natural sweetness and a creamy texture to the smoothie.

4. Creamy Greek Yogurt: Spoon in the Greek yogurt, adding a luscious creaminess to the smoothie while also contributing protein and probiotics.

5. A Touch of Sweetness: Drizzle honey or maple syrup into the blender to enhance the sweetness. Adjust the amount based on your desired level of sweetness. The natural sweetness from the fruits might be sufficient.

6. Hydrating Liquid: Pour in the coconut water or orange juice. The liquid will help blend the ingredients smoothly and enhance the tropical flavor. Choose coconut water for a more tropical taste or orange juice for a zesty twist.

7. Zesty Kick (Optional): If you enjoy a zesty kick, add the grated fresh ginger to the mix. The ginger will add a subtle zing to the smoothie.

8. Chill It Down: For a refreshing and cool smoothie, you can add a few ice cubes to the blender before blending.

9. Blend to a Tropical Fusion: Secure the blender's lid and blend all the ingredients until they combine into a smooth and tropical delight.
10. Taste and Enhance: After blending, take a moment to taste the Papaya Passion Smoothie. Adjust sweetness, ginger, or flavors as needed to suit your taste preferences.
11. Serve and Garnish: Pour the tropical elixir into a glass and garnish with fresh mint leaves, if desired. The mint leaves will add an extra touch of freshness and visual appeal.
12. Savor the Papaya Passion: Grab a straw and savor every sip of this exotic and revitalizing creation.

The Papaya Passion Smoothie is more than just a blend of fruits; it's a tropical escape into a world of delightful flavors. As you enjoy the tropical sweetness and zesty freshness of this exotic creation, embrace the goodness of papaya, pineapple, and banana. Let this smoothie be your refreshing and revitalizing journey to a tropical paradise. Cheers to the passion of Papaya Passion Smoothie!

Recipe Fourteen: Cherry Almond Cream Smoothie

Ingredients:

- ✓ 1 cup fresh or frozen cherries (pitted)
- ✓ 1 cup unsweetened almond milk
- ✓ 1 ripe banana
- ✓ 1/4 cup plain Greek yogurt
- ✓ 1 tablespoon almond butter
- ✓ 1 tablespoon honey or maple syrup (adjust for desired sweetness)
- ✓ 1/2 teaspoon almond extract
- ✓ 1/4 teaspoon vanilla extract
- ✓ Ice cubes (optional, for a chilled smoothie)

Instructions:

1. Prepare the Cherries: If using fresh cherries, wash them thoroughly and remove the pits. If using frozen cherries, allow them to thaw slightly.
2. Peel and Prepare the Banana: Peel the ripe banana and break it into chunks. The banana will provide natural sweetness and a creamy texture to the smoothie.
3. Creamy Greek Yogurt: Add the plain Greek yogurt to the blender. The yogurt will contribute a luscious creaminess and boost the smoothie's protein content.

4. Nutty Almond Butter: Spoon in the almond butter. The almond butter will enrich the smoothie with nutty flavor and healthy fats.
5. A Touch of Sweetness: Drizzle honey or maple syrup into the blender to enhance the sweetness. Adjust the amount based on your desired level of sweetness. The natural sweetness from the fruits might be sufficient.
6. Almond and Vanilla Extracts: Add the almond extract and vanilla extract to the mix. These extracts will add a delightful aroma and depth of flavor to the smoothie.
7. Creamy Almond Milk: Pour in the unsweetened almond milk. The almond milk will create a creamy and nutty base for the smoothie.
8. Chill It Down: For a refreshing and cool smoothie, you can add a few ice cubes to the blender before blending.
9. Blend to a Creamy Bliss: Secure the blender's lid and blend all the ingredients until they combine into a smooth and creamy delight.
10. Taste and Adjust: After blending, take a moment to taste the Cherry Almond Cream Smoothie. Adjust sweetness or flavors as needed to suit your taste preferences.

11. Serve and Enjoy: Pour the luscious elixir into a glass and enjoy the creamy and nutty goodness with every delightful sip.

The Cherry Almond Cream Smoothie is more than just a blend of fruits and nuts; it's a creamy and indulgent treat. As you relish the sweet-tart flavor and nutty creaminess of this delightful creation, embrace the goodness of cherries, almond butter, and almond extract. Let this smoothie be your comforting and satisfying escape into a world of rich and creamy flavors. Cheers to the creamy delight of Cherry Almond Cream Smoothie!

Recipe Fifteen: Ginger Turmeric Twist Smoothie

Ingredients:

- ✓ 1 cup chopped fresh pineapple
- ✓ 1 ripe banana
- ✓ 1 teaspoon grated fresh ginger
- ✓ 1/2 teaspoon grated fresh turmeric (or 1/4 teaspoon ground turmeric)
- ✓ 1 cup unsweetened coconut water or water
- ✓ 1 tablespoon honey or maple syrup (adjust for desired sweetness)
- ✓ 1/2 teaspoon ground cinnamon
- ✓ A pinch of black pepper (optional, to enhance turmeric's benefits)
- ✓ Ice cubes (optional, for a chilled smoothie)

Instructions:

1. Prep the Pineapple: Start by chopping the fresh pineapple into bite-sized pieces. The sweet and tangy pineapple will be the star of this vibrant smoothie.
2. Peel and Prepare the Banana: Peel the ripe banana and add it to the blender. The banana will provide natural sweetness and a creamy texture to the smoothie.
3. Grate the Ginger and Turmeric: Grate the fresh ginger and turmeric directly into the

blender. Both ginger and turmeric will add a zesty and warm twist to the smoothie, along with their numerous health benefits.

4. Sweetness of Your Choice: Drizzle honey or maple syrup into the blender to enhance the sweetness. Adjust the amount based on your desired level of sweetness.
5. Hydrating Liquid: Pour in the unsweetened coconut water or water. The liquid will help blend the ingredients smoothly and add a tropical touch if using coconut water.
6. Cinnamon Spice: Sprinkle the ground cinnamon into the mix. The warm and comforting spice will complement the ginger and turmeric, adding a delightful aroma and flavor.
7. Black Pepper Boost (Optional): For enhanced turmeric benefits, add a pinch of black pepper. The black pepper aids in the absorption of turmeric's active compound, curcumin.
8. Chill It Down: For a refreshing and cool smoothie, you can add a few ice cubes to the blender before blending.
9. Blend to a Vibrant Twist: Secure the blender's lid and blend all the ingredients until they combine into a smooth and vibrant twist.

10. Taste and Enhance: After blending, take a moment to taste the Ginger Turmeric Twist Smoothie. Adjust sweetness, spices, or flavors as needed to suit your taste preferences.
11. Serve and Enjoy: Pour the invigorating elixir into a glass and enjoy the zesty and warming goodness with every revitalizing sip.

The Ginger Turmeric Twist Smoothie is more than just a blend of fruits and spices; it's a zesty and nourishing delight. As you enjoy the tropical sweetness and warming spices of this flavorful creation, embrace the goodness of ginger, turmeric, and cinnamon. Let this smoothie be your revitalizing and flavorful escape into a world of vibrant and aromatic delights. Cheers to the zesty twist of Ginger Turmeric Twist Smoothie!

Recipe Sixteen: Blueberry Walnut Wonder Smoothie

Ingredients:

- ✓ 1 cup fresh or frozen blueberries
- ✓ 1 ripe banana
- ✓ 1/4 cup walnuts
- ✓ 1 cup unsweetened almond milk (or any milk of your choice)
- ✓ 1 tablespoon honey or maple syrup (adjust for desired sweetness)
- ✓ 1/2 teaspoon vanilla extract
- ✓ A pinch of ground cinnamon
- ✓ Ice cubes (optional, for a chilled smoothie)

Instructions:

1. Blueberry Bliss: If using fresh blueberries, rinse them under cool water. If using frozen blueberries, allow them to thaw slightly. The sweet and antioxidant-rich blueberries will be the star of this delightful smoothie.
2. Peel and Prepare the Banana: Peel the ripe banana and add it to the blender. The banana will provide natural sweetness and a creamy texture to the smoothie.
3. Nutty Walnuts: Add the walnuts to the blender. The walnuts will add a delightful

nutty flavor and boost the smoothie's omega-3 fatty acids content.

4. A Touch of Sweetness: Drizzle honey or maple syrup into the blender to enhance the sweetness. Adjust the amount based on your desired level of sweetness.

5. Creamy Liquid: Pour in the unsweetened almond milk (or any milk of your choice). The milk will create a creamy and smooth consistency for the smoothie.

6. Vanilla Essence: Add the vanilla extract to the mix. The vanilla will add a pleasant aroma and depth of flavor to the smoothie.

7. Warmth of Cinnamon: Sprinkle the ground cinnamon into the blender. The warm and comforting spice will complement the blueberries and add a delightful touch to the smoothie.

8. Chill It Down: For a refreshing and cool smoothie, you can add a few ice cubes to the blender before blending.

9. Blend to a Nutty Wonder: Secure the blender's lid and blend all the ingredients until they combine into a smooth and nutty wonder.

10. Taste and Adjust: After blending, take a moment to taste the Blueberry Walnut Wonder Smoothie. Adjust sweetness or

flavors as needed to suit your taste
preferences.

11. Serve and Savor: Pour the nutty elixir into a
glass and enjoy the wholesome goodness
with every delightful sip.

The Blueberry Walnut Wonder Smoothie is more than just a blend of fruits and nuts; it's a wholesome and nutritious delight. As you relish the sweet-tart flavor and nutty creaminess of this delightful creation, embrace the goodness of blueberries and walnuts. Let this smoothie be your comforting and satisfying escape into a world of rich and wholesome flavors. Cheers to the wonder of Blueberry Walnut Wonder Smoothie!

Recipe Seventeen: Mango Carrot Kick Smoothie

Ingredients:

- ✓ 1 ripe mango (peeled, pitted, and chopped)
- ✓ 1 large carrot (peeled and chopped)
- ✓ 1 ripe banana
- ✓ 1 cup orange juice (freshly squeezed or store-bought)
- ✓ 1/2 cup plain Greek yogurt (low-fat or non-fat)
- ✓ 1 tablespoon honey or maple syrup (adjust for desired sweetness)
- ✓ 1/2 teaspoon grated fresh ginger
- ✓ Ice cubes (optional, for a chilled smoothie)
- ✓ Fresh mint leaves for garnish (optional)

Instructions:

1. Prepare the Mango and Carrot: Start by peeling the ripe mango, removing the pit, and chopping the flesh into small pieces. Peel the large carrot and chop it into smaller chunks.
2. Peel and Prepare the Banana: Peel the ripe banana and add it to the blender. The banana will provide natural sweetness and a creamy texture to the smoothie.
3. Creamy Greek Yogurt: Add the plain Greek yogurt to the blender. The yogurt will

contribute a luscious creaminess and boost the smoothie's protein content.

4. A Touch of Sweetness: Drizzle honey or maple syrup into the blender to enhance the sweetness. Adjust the amount based on your desired level of sweetness.

5. Zesty Ginger: Grate the fresh ginger directly into the blender. The ginger will add a zesty and invigorating kick to the smoothie.

6. Vibrant Orange Juice: Pour in the orange juice. The orange juice will provide a tangy and citrusy base for the smoothie.

7. Chill It Down: For a refreshing and cool smoothie, you can add a few ice cubes to the blender before blending.

8. Blend to a Zingy Kick: Secure the blender's lid and blend all the ingredients until they combine into a smooth and zingy kick.

9. Taste and Adjust: After blending, take a moment to taste the Mango Carrot Kick Smoothie. Adjust sweetness, ginger, or flavors as needed to suit your taste preferences.

10. Serve and Garnish: Pour the zesty elixir into a glass and garnish with fresh mint leaves, if desired. The mint leaves will add an extra touch of freshness and visual appeal.

11. Savor the Mango Carrot Kick: Grab a straw and savor every sip of this zesty and invigorating creation.

The Mango Carrot Kick Smoothie is more than just a blend of fruits and veggies; it's a zingy and refreshing delight. As you enjoy the tropical sweetness and zesty kick of this flavorful creation, embrace the goodness of mango, carrot, and ginger. Let this smoothie be your revitalizing and energizing escape into a world of vibrant and wholesome flavors. Cheers to the kick of Mango Carrot Kick Smoothie!

Recipe Eighteen: Raspberry Cocoa Delight Smoothie

Ingredients:

- ✓ 1 cup fresh or frozen raspberries
- ✓ 1 ripe banana
- ✓ 1 tablespoon unsweetened cocoa powder
- ✓ 1 cup unsweetened almond milk (or any milk of your choice)
- ✓ 1 tablespoon honey or maple syrup (adjust for desired sweetness)
- ✓ 1/2 teaspoon pure vanilla extract
- ✓ A pinch of salt
- ✓ Ice cubes (optional, for a chilled smoothie)
- ✓ Dark chocolate shavings or cocoa nibs for garnish (optional)

Instructions:

1. Raspberry Bliss: If using fresh raspberries, rinse them under cool water. If using frozen raspberries, allow them to thaw slightly. The sweet-tart raspberries will be the star of this delightful smoothie.
2. Peel and Prepare the Banana: Peel the ripe banana and add it to the blender. The banana

will provide natural sweetness and a creamy
texture to the smoothie.

3. Cocoa Magic: Add the unsweetened cocoa powder to the blender. The cocoa powder will add a rich chocolate flavor and turn this smoothie into a delightful cocoa delight.

4. A Touch of Sweetness: Drizzle honey or maple syrup into the blender to enhance the sweetness. Adjust the amount based on your desired level of sweetness.

5. Creamy Liquid: Pour in the unsweetened almond milk (or any milk of your choice). The milk will create a creamy and smooth consistency for the smoothie.

6. Pure Vanilla: Add the pure vanilla extract to the mix. The vanilla will add a delightful aroma and complement the chocolate flavor.

7. A Pinch of Salt: Add a pinch of salt to enhance the flavors and balance the sweetness of the smoothie.

8. Chill It Down: For a refreshing and cool smoothie, you can add a few ice cubes to the blender before blending.

9. Blend to a Cocoa Delight: Secure the blender's lid and blend all the ingredients until they combine into a smooth and luscious cocoa delight.

10. Taste and Adjust: After blending, take a moment to taste the Raspberry Cocoa Delight Smoothie. Adjust sweetness or flavors as needed to suit your taste preferences.
11. Serve and Garnish: Pour the chocolaty elixir into a glass and garnish with dark chocolate shavings or cocoa nibs, if desired. The garnish will add an extra touch of decadence and visual appeal.
12. Savor the Raspberry Cocoa Delight: Grab a straw and savor every sip of this rich and delightful creation.

The Raspberry Cocoa Delight Smoothie is more than just a blend of fruits and chocolate; it's a decadent and indulgent treat. As you enjoy the sweet-tart raspberries and rich cocoa flavor of this flavorful creation, embrace the goodness of berries and chocolate. Let this smoothie be your comforting and satisfying escape into a world of rich and delightful flavors. Cheers to the delight of Raspberry Cocoa Delight Smoothie!